Waxing For Women

~

The Subtle Art of Waxing

By

Sarah H. Carter

Table of Contents

ISBN-13: 978-1548045791
ISBN-10: 1548045799

Foreword

Everybody loves a flawless skin: blemish-free, clear, smooth, and for some areas, also hairless. The desire for this level of beauty is observable in both men and women but more apparent in the fairer sex. Hair removal among women has been an acceptable and regular hygiene practice for some. The commonality of hair removal is apparent in the number of ways that it can be done personally or availed from wellness centers. One of the common, convenient, and more popular hair removal services is waxing.

Different types of hair removal

Shaving

Shaving is a hair removal technique using a blade through razors or electric shavers to trim the hair short. It only deals with the visible hair shaft over the skin and does not remove the hair from its root.

Shaving is done only on wet skin. One may first soap the area until bubbles and foam cover it. A shaving cream, which can also be in foam form may be applied prior to shaving.

Shaving does not affect hair thickness, color, or growth rate contrary to popular belief. The shaved area may be washed with soap and rinsed with water after the procedure. After washing, the shaved area is pat dry and an anti-inflammatory cream may be applied after to soothe the shaved area and prevent further redness, swelling, or irritation.

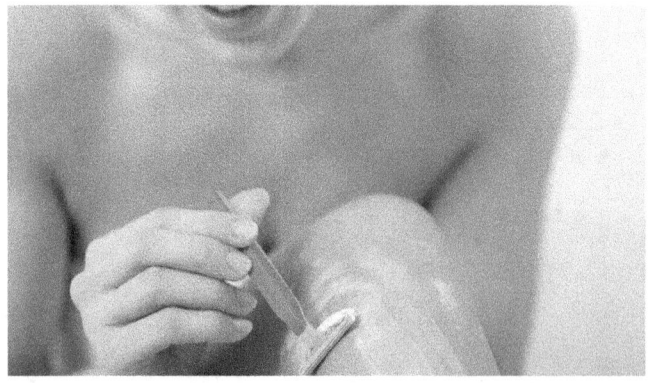

Depilatory cream

Depilatories can be highly alkaline or acidic in formulation. They work by dissolving the hair, which one can just rinse off after application. As depilatories work mainly through some chemical reaction, it is advised to first have them tested on your skin like the back of your hand or forearm for any allergic reactions like itchiness, redness, swelling, and the like.

Depilatories similarly work like shaving as these products only deal with the shaft of the hair and not its roots. Techniques or products like such allow for quick regrowth of hair so you may have to shave or use a depilatory cream more often than other methods that remove the hair up to its roots.

Unless you have some sensitivity to the product, depilatories are usually painless at any point of use. Depilatories do not usually leave adverse effects on skin which it is compatible with except for some odd smell. There are however many formulations on the market that try to go around this by creating scented ones.

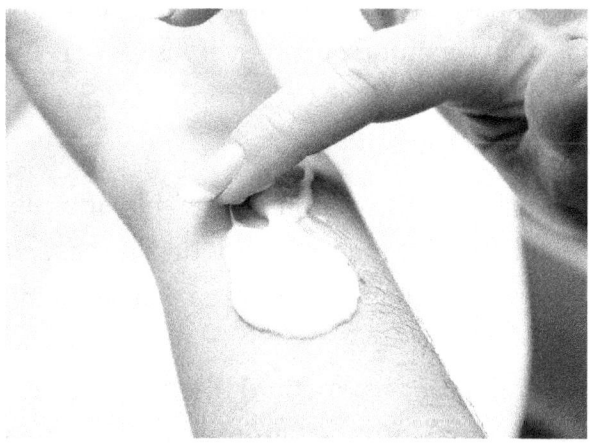

Laser

Laser hair removal is among the techniques that you can avail as a service from a dermatology clinic or wellness center with trained personnel. The laser method mainly uses heat to destroy hair up to its follicles. Anesthetic cream or gels may be applied to the target area prior to treatment in order to protect the skin from laser and to reduce or remove pain during the procedure.

Before signing up for sessions, remember to check on the license and training of the personnel who will perform the laser treatment on you. Laser hair removal is considered as a medical procedure and dermatologists, licensed doctors, and trained personnel are the only people who can perform this service.

As for the actual procedures on laser hair removal, preparatory steps such as trimming your hair and adjusting the laser intensity may be done aside from applying protective gels or cream on the target area.

The laser treatment may feel tingly as it is an actual zapping of high heat light on your hair, which is after all rooted on your skin and has pain receptors. Moreover, as laser is intense light, you and the technician may also need to wear eye protection throughout the treatment.

After the treatment, anti-inflammatory gels, lotions, or cream, ice pack, or cold water may be provided to ease any pain or discomfort on the newly treated area. Laser hair treatments are among the most expensive options and are usually available as packages. This method also involves returning for a number of sessions until the hair does not regrow anymore.

Electrolysis

Electrolysis hair removal is another hassle-free method yielding permanent hair loss that one can avail from a trained electronologist. Electrolysis is a method that uses a fine needle to reach the hair follicle where light current or high heat is introduced to destroy the hair root. The hair removal procedure is completed by using tweezers to pick the rootless hairs.

Electrolysis can be done on other body parts such as the abdomen, breasts, eyebrows, face, legs, and thighs. Each session may last from fifteen (15) to sixty (60) minutes (1 hour) depending on the hair volume. Achieving complete hair loss does not also have a set number of required sessions and may vary from person to person depending on hair growth rate. Just like laser treatment, electrolysis may be slightly painful but can be controlled with topical anesthesia.

A high skilled professional should be the one to administer the treatment. Electrolysis is also more expensive compared to other hair removal procedures.

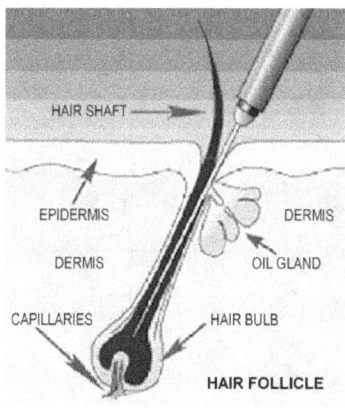

Tweezing

Tweezing, also known as plucking, is a mechanical hair removal technique done with tweezers or metal forceps, which are slender and small pincer-like tools that you can use to pick or pinch and pull hair from its roots.

Tweezing is probably the most inexpensive hair removal method but it does require more patience. Tweezing is mostly used to shape the eyebrows and remove stray hairs from the face. This technique may also be done after waxing to get rid of smaller or thinner stray hair. We also mentioned earlier that tweezing is also done after electrolysis to pick the rootless hairs. Some also use tweezing to remove underarm hair.

This hair removal technique may consume a lot of time and cause more pain weigh against other techniques. It does not really kill the hair follicles and so hair just keeps regrowing after some time and the same way it was. Tweezing may also result to ingrown hairs, scarring, or pitting.

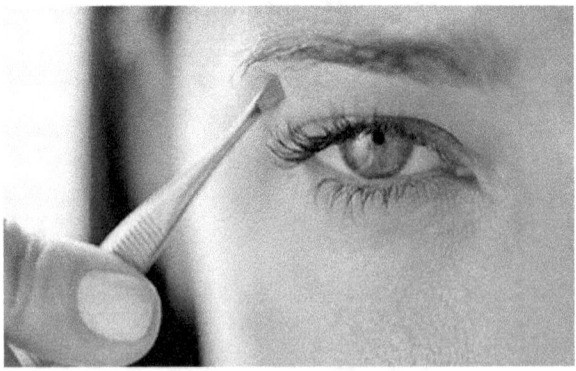

Waxing

Waxing is a hair removal technique that one can either personally do or avail in salons. Waxing has similar hair removing mechanisms with tweezing. This method basically removes hair by pulling it from its roots. However, instead of manually picking the hair one by one, waxing is able to remove hair from a patch by using wax as a form of adhesive that sticks hair into a strip. One can pull against the hair growth direction at once, uprooting many hairs in one go.

Waxing results can keep hair away longer than shaving as it removes the hair follicles. There is no risk of scarring or nicking yourself with this technique. It is fast, convenient, and with many people offering this service, its price has also been cost-effective these days. When availed in salons, waxing can also be hassle-free. For many people, waxing is able to lessen hair growth and slow hair growth rate. Repeated waxing may also lead to regrowth of finer hair.

Waxing can be done in different body parts including the underarms, legs, face, and even the bikini area. Waxing is a highly flexible procedure that one can further optimize for convenience and maximized results.

The rest of this guide will discuss further details on waxing including the different kinds of wax used for procedures, the materials, available kits for home-use, waxing tips, preparations, and troubleshooting.

Different kinds of waxing

Strip waxing (soft wax)

Strip waxing is named as such because it uses strips where soft wax can stick to. Soft wax is a stickier type of wax. It needs prior heating until it achieves softer consistency that can be applied over the skin in the same direction of hair growth. Strips are then put on top of the applied wax and left there until it hardens. Later on, the strips are pulled off in the opposite direction of hair growth. The efficiency of using soft wax lies more on the speed when pulling the wax and not just on how long or how hard the wax has dried. Soft wax is also not very effective on ingrown hair.

When using soft wax, it is advisable to have at least ¼ inch of hair growth. This gives the wax enough hair length to cling on making it easier to pull. Soft wax is also recommended to use on larger areas like the back, legs, and arms. To prepare the skin, it is cleansed first and powder is applied over the area. The powder dries up extra moisture on the skin and protects it from the melted soft wax. Applying powder may be necessary because soft wax is sticky enough to cling to the skin itself and can hurt when pulled. Powder application prevents this interaction.

Soft wax can have a creamy base or even honey. Some formulations may be scented and have other ingredients that help the skin to recover or prevent pain. Different types of wax are also available.

Pre-made strips

This type consists of wax on a strip. Most can be pre-heated by just rubbing them between one's palms. They are convenient to use and are easily available. There is also enough wax spread evenly on the strip so you do not have to worry about over or under spreading of soft wax. Some strips may be used more than once depending on the area being treated.

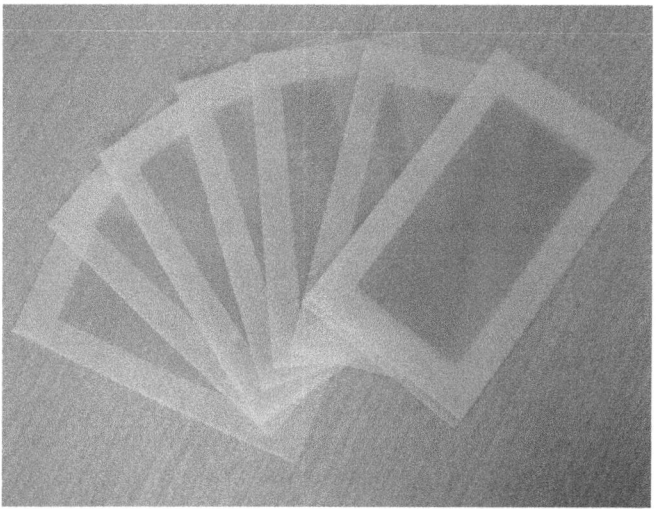

Heated soft wax

It can be heated through a warmer or a microwave. The heat makes the wax spreadable and even softens the hair and skin reducing pain when pulled off.

Cold soft wax

Soft wax can also be applied without pre-heating. However, this method makes the soft wax harder to apply and more painful when removed. It is a more convenient method because it skips the pre-heating but is also more prone to leave hair behind when applied unevenly or improperly.

Strip-less waxing (hard wax)

Strip-less waxing gets rid of the strip to assist in pulling off wax applied on the skin. This method uses hard wax, which can be applied cold, in room temperature, or pre-heated, and just peeled off after cooling and hardening.

Since hard wax hardens well, it acquires the tendency to break when applied to large areas. It is then usually applied in smaller areas with more sensitive skin like the bikini area, ear, face nose, and even underarms. Hard wax is also able to adhere well to hair and can handle both ingrown and fine hair.

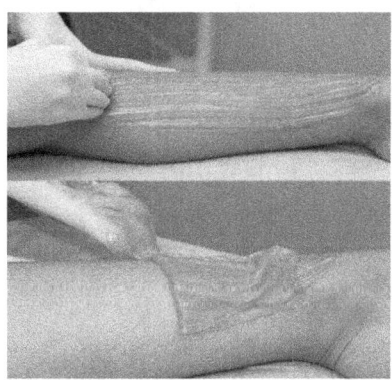

Preparing for hard waxing can be done by first applying oil or powder on the target area. Hard wax is then heated, cooled down a bit, then applied evenly and more thickly than soft wax over the skin. It is left to rest until it can be peeled off. This method can still hurt like other hair removal techniques but people generally find this method less painful as hard wax does not pull skin unlike soft wax. Treatments are finished off by rinsing with water and by applying anti-inflammatory creams or gels.

Persian waxing (sugaring wax)

Persian waxing is also known as sugar waxing or sugaring. It got its other names from the sugar mixture it uses for hair removal in place of actual wax. The sugar mixture may also include water, lemon, cornstarch, molasses, and even honey. It is usually boiled until thick and may be used after cooled down in lukewarm or room temperatures.

Sugaring wax is found to be a less painful substitute to wax as the mixture does not stick to the skin. As aforementioned, wax, particularly soft wax, can get sticky and messy as it adheres to skin (due to resin components). This presents the tendency of wax to also pull skin that can hurt. Sugar waxing is also available in cooler temperatures, which reduce the risk of burning when used.

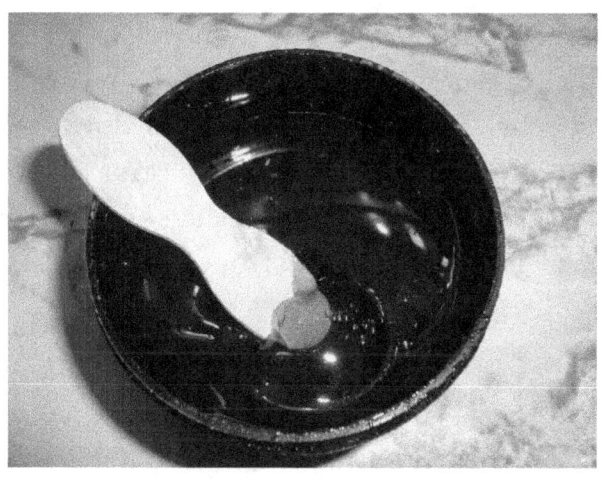

Professional sugar wax usually contains additional wax aside from sugar mixture. As for homemade sugaring wax, recipes are available online. The addition of lemon is important when preparing sugar mix. It is added for its acidity, which breaks down the glucose and fructose in the mixture as similarly observed in candy-making. This step then gives the sugaring wax its amorphous or non-crystalline form that can be easily applied on skin even when cooled.

Sugar waxing is a hair removal technique practiced even before, mostly in Persia and other Middle Eastern countries that even probably used honey as the original mixture base. Sugar wax uses natural ingredients and homemade ones can be relatively cheap to make. Some very sensitive skin may however remain irritated by the sugar though it is generally hypoallergenic. This reaction may be avoided by taking antihistamine prior to the sugaring treatment.

Sugaring can be an efficient hair removal treatment. It does not harm the skin and removes even ingrown hair. It is simply applied over the skin and waited to cool down and harden. Powder may also be applied on the area prior to spreading the wax to assure that the skin is dry. The sugar wax then traps hair as it hardens and pulls them from its roots when lifted.

Sugar wax does not stick to skin so much that it can hurt, but its stickiness is enough to also exfoliate the skin lightly by lifting dead skin cells. After sugaring, the skin can be easily cleansed and other remaining mixtures can be removed by simply rinsing with water. Sugaring can be done on the face, underarms, back, legs, and even on the bikini area.

Waxing supplies

Regular waxing kits

(strips) → legs and underarms

People get rid of unwanted hair on the legs and underarms. With this demand, many products on the market are then made available for these purposes.

People who do not have the time to study more complex procedures, who do not want bulky equipment, and want simple and clean methods usually just opt for regular waxing kits with strips.

Strip waxing kits may come in variety as well. More common forms come in strips with pre-applied wax on them already. These strips are pre-heated in some way, usually by rubbing between one's palms before using. Once the wax on the strip is softened, it is then laid over the unwanted hair following its growth. The strip is left for a while until it cools and hardens, and then pulled off against the direction of hair growth. Some strips can be reused a few times though they may have trouble removing ingrown or fine hair.

Another variation of waxing kits that use strips can also use wax in cream form placed in a separate tube or port. These kits usually come with applicator sticks that help you apply and spread the creamy or soft wax on the desired area. Depending if the wax still needs to be pre-heated, such kits may already have heating equipment with them.

Some products are already creamy in room temperature and you may apply them right away without pre-heating. These creams just harden later on after application. A strip is placed on the softened or creamy wax before it is allowed to dry. Once cooled and hardened, the strip is then pulled the same way pre-made strips are lifted off from the skin.

Aside from the main waxing materials, other strip kits provide pre- and /or post-waxing strips, wipes, creams, gels, or powders that can help in promoting the adhesion between hair and the wax or reduce pain and inflammation from the process.

Hard waxing kits

(strip less) → bikini area

Microwaveable Kits

If you are only planning to wax small areas then microwaveable kits may be the way to go. Greater amounts of wax may still be heated through a microwave while placed in a wax but this does not ensure even heating throughout the whole amount. Unevenly heated wax presents a risk of burns and so it might be advisable to stick to smaller amounts of wax for these kits.

Microwaveable kits usually have bars or tablets or hard wax plus a number of applicators. The waxes may vary in color and may sometimes even have other ingredients to help with skin care or pain reduction during the waxing.

On the other hand, applicators may vary in material, size, and number. Some kits may only provide one applicator per size, while others mostly for wax warmers (read below), and may include several ones to avoid the need of double-dipping.

Applicators are also usually made of wood that looks like reshaped and resized Popsicle sticks. Applicator size varies to correspond to the body areas that it will cover. Larger applicators are for the legs and back while medium ones may be used for the armpits and bikini area. The smallest ones are probably used on the face for the eyebrows or upper lip. Wax cans may also be provided in some microwaveable kits. If not, wax cans may be bought separately instead.

Wax Warmers

If you plan to maintain a waxing habit including large areas, then it is advisable to consider investing on a wax warmer. Wax warmers evenly heat wax in a wax can compared to microwaves. Some wax warmers may only have an on and off switch while others provide more control by having temperature adjustment options. Salons or spas generally rely on wax warmers for their services as using so proves to be highly convenient.

In addition to controlling for temperature, wax warmers also maintain the wax warm. You do not have to reheat. There is also lesser chance of overheating especially for those with temperature controls.

Despite the flexibility on temperature control, remember that the amount of wax being heated affects how much heat the amount can contain. Smaller amounts of wax will heat up faster and are prone to overheating while ample amounts of wax are evenly heated in general.

Kits that include wax warmers may also provide accessory materials for pre- and post-skin care. The variety of hard wax and applicators for microwaveable kits are also observed for kits including wax warmers.

Persian waxing kits

We have mentioned before that Persian or sugar wax can be easily used even in cool or room temperature. Before, Persian waxing kits usually just have the cold wax and an applicator stick. It may have several applicator sticks and pre and post-skin care accessories, too.

Though it is advisable to buy better quality, professional grade waxes, it is also possible to come up with your own Persian or sugaring kit. Recipes on sugar wax can be easily found on the internet and the ingredients it uses are all natural and are mostly found in your pantry. Applicator sticks may be substituted by Popsicle sticks or spatula-like applicators.

Waxing tips

Use baby powder before waxing

We have been mentioning the use of powder before applying wax on skin. This is to fully dry the skin and create a barrier between it and the wax.

Avoid burning yourself with the hot wax

Some waxes need to be fully melted before application and these require steps to melting the wax in high temperatures. Wax works the same way at lower temperature though and you do not have to endure being burned to remove your hair. Follow the instructions when you buy products that require heating.

Allow pre-heated wax to cool as well. What feels warm for your palms or other thick-skinned parts will feel extremely hot for other areas (e.g. pubic region). The extreme temperatures can even take some of your skin off if not only burn it.

If you are still unsure about the temperature of the wax for other body parts, you can test it first on lesser sensitive areas like the back of your hand or at your wrist. Apply some wax on it and see if you can tolerate its current temperature. Do not use a thermometer on wax as it may only stick on it.

Make sure you have long enough hair

Wax needs to have enough hair length to cling on to before it can perform its wonders. Wax cannot cling on hair that is too short. On the other hand, having too long hair might make it more painful because of too much pull force. Salons have their personnel trained for this and may just do the trimming if you avail waxing outside your home. You should have at least 1/8 of an inch.

Do not wax the same area twice

Most waxes are pre-heated by melting them in high temperatures. Waxing an area and placing another batch of warm wax on the newly waxed spot may then only irritate the open pores of the area and cause redness or swelling. Unless you are using pre-made strips that can be reused for several times, do not wax the same area twice especially if it involves applying substances again on the newly waxed area.

Consider a numbing cream

As mentioned, all of us have different levels for pain tolerance. Another way to prevent the pain from waxing is by applying a numbing cream on the area prior to waxing. These creams are left for a period of time and may last up to 30 minutes. Some spas and salons sell and/ or include such cream in their shop or services.

Some wax can be molten in the microwave

There are many ways to pre-heat wax. Some pre-made strips just require rubbing from between your palms while other kits already provide heating ports for your convenience. Other products may also allow using the microwave but be sure to read the product's instructions carefully when doing so. Make sure you follow the microwave conditions needed (e.g. time in microwave, temperature set) for the wax to melt well.

Apply pressure against the skin

Some pressure can help soothe the pain, much more reduce any bleeding from the newly opened pores. Just make sure your hand is clean. Salons usually have their personnel wear gloves during waxing. Make sure these are new ones. Also, check if the rest of the area and the materials are clean.

Don't wax before or during your period

Hormonal changes that occur in the female body during menstruation can affect the body's general sensitivity to any sensation especially for pain. Check your cycle schedule. As much as possible, only schedule waxing after your monthly period. Waxing before one's period must also be followed strictly for those planning to do it in their bikini area to avoid infections. Remember that waxing opens up pores when it uproots hair so it is best to keep the waxed area dry and free from contamination for quite some time after the treatment.

Do not drink alcohol or caffeine before waxing

Alcohol and caffeine both boost hormones in the blood that increase one's sensitivity to sensations just as how periods do it naturally. It is therefore advised that you avoid caffeinated food and beverages that can spike up the hormones and make you more sensitive to pain.

Before you wax

Do not wax when you have broken skin or inflammation

Any form of opening in the skin such as wounds, burns, cuts, or open pores can be a gateway to infectious microorganisms. Similarly, irritated and inflamed skin cannot tolerate further disturbance until they have soothed off. Waxing must then be done only on dry, clean, and intact skin to avoid infections and further worsening of skin conditions.

Prepare a soothing cream or lotion

Find a non-irritating and light lotion and put it in the fridge to cool the night before you wax. Once your waxing is over and your skin has started to recover a bit, you may apply this pre-cooled lotion to soothe any pain or discomfort from your freshly bare armpits, legs, or face spots.

Light exfoliate. No harsh scrubs

To promote adhesion only between wax and hair, light exfoliation may also be done prior to waxing. Light exfoliation means that you only aim to remove dead skin cells. Too much scrubbing can irritate the skin. It can also lead to broken skin if scrubbing is done harshly. As aforementioned, waxing must not be done on broken and/ or irritated skin.

Moisturize your skin some DAYS BEFORE waxing

Moisturizing your skin is generally a good practice and advisable even prior to waxing. Moisturizing is recommended until the actual day of your waxing as healthy and well-moisturized hair allows the wax to be lifted off easily from the skin during waxing. However, too much moisturizing and doing it just before waxing interfere with the wax's grip on the hair.

The waxing process

Cleanse the area. You may wash off the area with soap and water then pat dry or use a very light and neutral astringent applied with cotton.

Apply anti-inflammatory product and /or powder. Consider applying pre-wax anti-inflammatory creams or gels first on the area to be waxed. Apply the powder next to make sure the area is dry and free of oils. This helps promote the adhesion between the wax and your hair.

Apply the wax. If using pre-made strips, pre-heat the strip between your palms and spread following the direction of hair growth. If you are using melted wax, use an applicator to spread the wax against the direction of hair growth. Do not over-apply the wax.

Wax off. Use your free hand to pull the skin without hair in the opposite direction you are pulling the strip or wax. This helps make the skin taut. Also, remember to pull off the wax in the opposite direction of hair growth and parallel to the skin (not upwards that might be your instinctive tendency).

Press the waxed area. This step helps ease the throbbing pain after waxing a specific area.

Repeat. Repeat the procedures for the other brow. If you are using pre-made strips, you may also wax the area again should you miss some hair strands.

Deal with missed hairs. If waxing again with pre-made strips cannot get rid of shorter missed hairs, use tweezers to pick the stray hairs off.

Remove remaining wax from the skin. You may use baby oil to remove remaining wax on your skin. If you underwent sugaring, water can cleanse off the remaining sugar wax.

Soothe the skin with post-wax products. Apply a cooling gel, Aloe Vera, or an anti-inflammatory gel or cream if available.

Above the Lip

Waxing your upper lip follows the general steps when waxing your other body parts. It is crucial to keep your skin clean to avoid any infections post-wax. Wash your face and remove any make-up or product applied on your skin. Use a facial cleanser to serve as an antiseptic to reduce the microbial load on your face as well. The face can be oily so make sure that you apply powder on your upper lip, too.

Use an applicator to spread wax in the same direction of your hair growth (i.e. downwards). Place a strip next if you are using soft wax or let the wax cool then peel off against the grain of hair growth if you are using hard wax. Apply pressure immediately after uprooting hair to dull the sting. Some suggests applying rubbing alcohol to cleanse the waxed area again. You may also use a cooling gel, aloe vera, or any other anti-inflammatory product to ease the pain and redness on the area.

Legs

The legs are among the larger areas that can be waxed, but the general steps in the waxing procedure similarly apply to these body parts. It is however important to consider that the legs may have longer and coarser hair than in other body parts. Make sure you have at least ¼ inch of hair length to optimize hair and wax adhesion. Also, remember to cleanse the area with an antiseptic prior to waxing.

Powder is also applied on the legs to promote hair and wax adhesion. Apply the wax following the direction of hair growth and pull or peel off the wax in the opposite direction. It is advisable to start in small patches especially if you are using hard wax as applying in large portions can break off the wax and result to poor hair removal.

Excess wax may be removed by oil or water for sugar wax. Anti-inflammatory gels or creams may also be applied post-wax. Make sure to avoid tight clothing (e.g. skinny jeans or any tight pants) as your skin tries to recover after waxing.

Underarms

The armpits are among the commonly waxed body parts and are considered to be one of the sensitive areas, too. The usual steps of cleansing and powdering are also applicable for the armpits. Applying wax can be trickier as there are different hair growth directions in the underarms. Check if certain patches change direction and apply the wax following hair growth. Once the wax has cooled, you may peel or pull it off against the direction of hair growth while keeping the skin taut with the other hand.

Anti-inflammatory gels, creams or oils may be applied after waxing. Do not apply deodorant or body sprays at least 24 hours after waxing. Some salons may even suggest not applying any product for at least several days. Also, avoid tight clothing while the skin recovers. After about three (3) days, consider lightly exfoliating your armpits to prevent ingrown hairs.

Bikini waxing

Bikini waxing is the hair removal process of the pubic area using wax. It can be done at home and is also offered in many salons. People go for a bikini wax for many different reasons including preference (i.e. they feel sexier without hair down there), hygienic purposes, work (i.e. for models), and fashion (i.e. for wearing bikini during summer).

Bikini waxing may entail more special considerations than when waxing other body parts. This area is definitely more sensitive and richer with microflora. There are however ways around these special cases to manage pain and avoid infections.

Pre-waxing

Do not schedule a wax before or during your period. Hormones shoot up during your period, which makes you more sensitive to pain. In addition, the bloody discharge from your menstruation can also get into your open pores after waxing that may lead to infections. Other ways to lessen the risks of infections include cleansing the area prior to waxing and keeping materials and area sanitary.

If you are availing a salon service, it is normal to feel conscious when exposing yourself down there to your waxologist, but rest assured that they have seen it all and won't judge you. Follow their instructions on how to position your legs no matter how awkward it may seem. An applicator will be used to apply the wax along the direction of your hair growth. Once cooled, the wax will be peeled or pulled off in the opposite direction.

If you are waxing on your own (though this is less encouraged), make sure that you are able to see your whole working area and that you are able to pull the skin taut when you finally pull off the wax.

Post-waxing

Tweezing may be done after waxing to deal with stray hairs that the wax missed. Once done with removing of all the hair, antiseptic and anti-inflammatory products can be applied on the waxed areas. Avoid wearing tight clothing and underwear to allow for the skin to breathe and to prevent sweating that can lead to infections. Also, do not apply any fragrant or chemically strong formulas on the waxed area within 24 hours of waxing.

Waxing Styles

American style
The American style, also known as "basic bikini", usually takes a triangle shape. It is done in consideration of the bikini swimwear and gets rid of the hair below the navel and at the sides of the inner thighs. Clients at a salon are usually asked to wear a bikini bottom to serve as a guide when doing the wax.

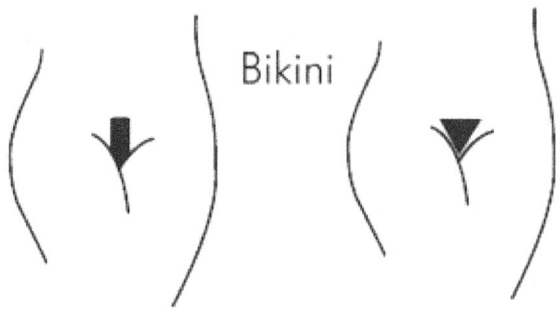

French style

The French style leaves lesser hair in the form of a strip aligned above the clitoris for more racy clothing that needs more skin exposed. The hair around the anus and the vulva may also be removed. Hard wax or soft wax strips may be used for this hair removal.

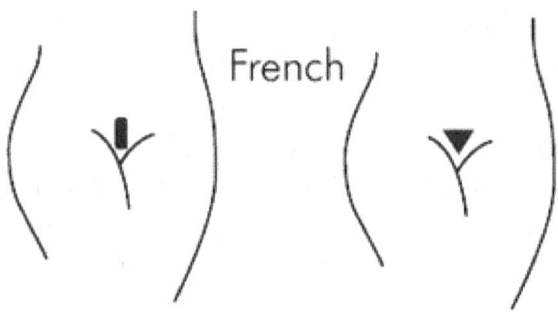

French

Brazilian style

The Brazilian style gets rid of all your hair below and even behind. You may be instructed by your waxologist to assume different positions to reach all these areas. Unlike the previous styles, Brazilian waxing requires one to bare it all. Hard wax is usually used for this style as in other bikini styles.

Brazilian

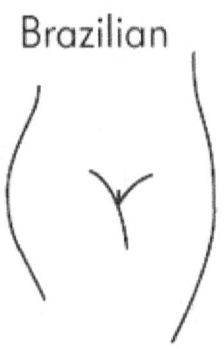

After the wax

Taking care of the skin

Cool shower

A warm shower helps open the pores prior to waxing, while a cool shower once the skin has rested, helps soothe the pain after the treatment. Make sure you take a bath only after at least 24 hours. This could change according to the advice from the salon and depending if you had other post-waxing substances applied after the treatment.

Moisturize every day

Since shaving removes the hair, it disrupts the oil production on the skin. Hairless skin is also less able to contain moisture and so other forms of skin rehydration may be necessary.

Be sure to only use a very light moisturizer on your skin and only after at least 24 hours post-treatment. Immediately applying products or other substances on your skin (unless it is an anti-inflammatory or soothing cream for post-waxing) is not recommended as it may only irritate the skin. Dead skin cells are likely to be lifted as well from waxing; moisturizing will help it recover.

Cooling gel

Pain may last only for a short time or longer depending on your skin's sensitivity. A cooling gel applied after waxing can be a good product to support your skin's recovery. Use it while you take other anti-inflammatory measures or stick to it as an alternative if you do not have the meds or those specialized soothing creams.

Exfoliate your skin

Once the pain and inflammation is over, you may now treat your skin like its old self. Exfoliate only after three (3) days post-waxing to avoid any irritation. This will get rid of dead skin cells that can get into your pores and clog them that may lead to ingrown hair.

Aloe Vera leaves have gel-like extract that you can apply to hydrate, moisturize, and soothe your skin. When using the plant, break off the leaf as close as possible to its base. Rinse the leaf with water to wash off any contaminant. Next, cut off the spikes on the edge of the leaf. Use a sharp knife to pass between the top and bottom layer of the leaf to extract the gel layer in between. Apply this gel on your skin directly.

No swimming or pool activities

Microorganisms like damp and wet areas. Keep your newly shaved areas dry unless applied with anti-inflammatory gels or creams. Avoid any swimming activities 24 hours after waxing. It can expose the open pores in your waxed area to possibly contaminated water as this may result to infections.

Take a pain reliever

If you are sensitive or it's your first time it might be better to take a pain reliever. There are a variety of over-the-counter pain relievers — Advil, aspirin, ibuprofen — for any type of pain including those caused by hair waxing. Take a pill at least thirty (30) minutes prior to your schedule to help minimize the pain ahead and/ or even after the treatment.

Use mineral based make-up to hide redness

If you had to wax unplanned and really need the post-wax redness and inflammation hidden for an event ahead, consider using mineral-based make-up, whether in foundation or concealer forms to temporarily hide your sore skin. Mineral-based make-up is finer and allows the skin to breathe, which lessens the risks of further irritation.

Things to avoid

There are many ways to irritate an already inflamed patch of skin. These include tight clothing, direct sunlight, and the application of any chemically-formulated substances on your waxed area within 24 hours of waxing. Tight clothing can lead to friction and sweating, which promotes infections. Direct sunlight can cause dark spots, and scented or alcohol-based formulas can redden and further irritate open pores.

Troubleshooting

Red bumps

Possible causes and Solutions:

- **Irritation**. Red bumps naturally occur right after waxing as the body's response to skin trauma (i.e. opening of pores by uprooting hair). These bumps are inflamed hair follicles. They usually go away on their own after a day or so. Cooling gels and cold compress may help in managing this kind of red bumps.

- **Folliculitis**. Sometimes, mild bacterial infection may occur on the waxed area and cause the hair follicles to swell into liquid-filled bumps. For sensitive skin, even friction or irritation can cause these red bumps. Folliculitis also usually just goes on on its own. For larger bumps that go with fever or similar symptoms, consult with your doctor.

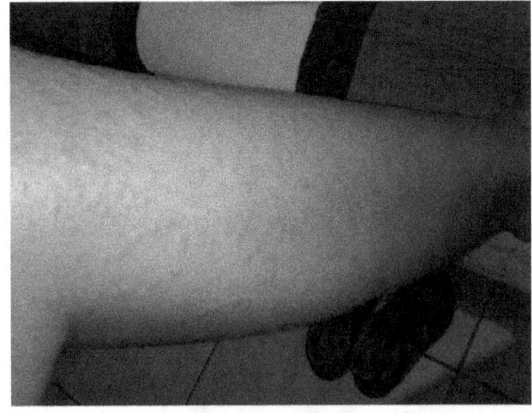

Ingrown hair

Also known as pseudofolliculitis, ingrown hair may later develop as red bumps on your recently waxed skin. Ingrown occurs when a regrowing hair curls back into the skin as it tries to shoot or emerge from the surface. Curly and coarse hair like those found in the armpits and underarms are those prone to ingrown. Exfoliate lightly at least three (3) days post-waxing to keep the skin free of dead skin cells that can interfere with regrowing hair.

Infections

Remember that waxing opens up one's pores when the hairs are uprooted. Open pores are similar to open wounds, which can be invaded by bacteria and other microorganisms. Remember to keep the skin free of contamination throughout the waxing process.

For pre-waxing, cleansing can be done by washing with soap and rinsing with water then patting dry or wiping off the skin with an astringent or antiseptic using a cotton ball.

During the waxing proper, make sure that you first wash your hands and have sanitary materials ready. When availing services from a salon, check their area first for cleanliness.

Special attention must also be given to the bikini area, another body part full of resident microflora. First off, make sure that you do not get your wax down there before and during your period. Periods do not only worsen the case when it comes to pain but discharges that go with it also bring microorganisms into open pores after waxing.

Additionally, avoid sexual activities after waxing your intimate area. As we were mentioning, open pores from waxing make one prone to infections including sexually transmitted diseases such as herpes and AIDS. You may think of using protection instead but touching or other form of stimulation may only irritate your currently sensitive skin and prolong the pain and inflammation at said area.

If you have infections immediately go to your local doctor and don't let it get worse.

Wax won't come off

Possible causes and solutions:

- **Skin is too dry**. When the waxed area is too dry, the skin's normal tendency is to absorb moisture from anything it gets in contact with next, which can possibly be the wax you applied. To avoid this, make sure you moisturize your skin days before waxing BUT NOT on the day itself as it will only make the area too moisturized instead. Doing so will interfere with the wax and hair adhesion.

- **Pulling too slow or too weakly**. Waxing is an inevitably painful process and slowing down the pull when waxing off is not really among the things you can do to manage the pain ahead. Pulling quick and steady is the key.

- **Wax applied is too thick**. For soft wax used with strips, a thin layer of wax is already enough to make the hair, wax, and strip adhere well with each other. Hard wax needs a little thicker layer but not so thick that it would be too difficult to peel off.

TIP: To clean up remaining wax, use oil for either hard or soft wax. Rinsing with water may be enough for sugar wax.

Hair does not come off

When waxing does not seem to work for you, retrace your steps to figure what you might be doing wrong. This problem is mostly due to poor adhesion between the hair and skin that might be affected by:

- **Skin condition**. When waxing, make sure that the area being waxed is clean and dry. Moisturize only on days before waxing and not hours prior to your schedule. Apply powder to remove other oils on the skin, which could interfere with the adhesion between the hair and your wax.

- **Hair length**. Also make sure that there is hair to adhere, too! Check the length of your hair. Generally, wax will fail to adhere well if the hair is too short. Keep it around ¼ inches long. There are, however, specialized waxes that may still adhere to microscopically small hair (which you can instead deal with tweezers). But wait, hair that is too long is not any better. At this other side of the extreme, hair might still come off or break off due to its length. Again, go for the right length (no need for a ruler though!).

- **Wax application**. Remember, spread along the direction of hair growth and pull off against hair growth direction. If you are using strips, make sure that you also spread it properly as wrinkles and folds will miss the hair.

- **Wax type**. Generally, hard wax is better for coarse hair. Strips are efficient on their own but may not have enough wax and strength for stronger hair so make sure you pick the appropriate wax depending on the area that you will be waxing.

Pimples

A pimple is another indication of contaminating a newly waxed area. Pimples can be prevented by keeping the waxing process sanitary all throughout. Exfoliate the skin lightly days before your wax. Cleanse the area prior to the treatment and consider using tea tree-based wax. Do not double-dip on the wax pot with the same applicator. After waxing, you may try to cleanse again by applying light witch hazel using a cotton ball. Prevent sweating by avoiding exercise and thick, tight clothing. By the time a pimple appears, never in any case should you pop it. Apply tea tree ointment or any of your usual pimple treatment products.

Bruising

It is important to apply ample force when pulling off your hair during your wax. However, in cases when the wax layer is too thick, the extra force applied may only lead to unwanted bruises in any body part and especially in the bikini area. Therefore, make sure you only apply a thick enough wax layer and pull or peel off the wax properly

Pain

Factors That Affect Pain Intensity and Ways to Control

- **Skin sensitivity and pain tolerance.** Each person is different with how much pain they can take. Women are said to have higher pain tolerance than men but that does not make women totally invincible. A woman's monthly period can affect their sensitivity to sensations including pain. Therefore, it is important that you schedule your waxing only after your period when your pain-promoting hormones are finally at bay.

  Alcohol and caffeine have the same hormone-promoting effects that lead to higher pain sensitivity. Avoiding food like coffee, tea, and soft drinks before and during your wax can help reduce pain during the treatment.

  If you are more inclined to depending on pills, it is also possible to manage pain by taking an anti-inflammatory before or after waxing. If planning to take prior treatment, pop a pill at least thirty (30) minutes before waxing.

Pre- and post-wax anti-inflammatory products in gel, cream, or oil forms are also available for one's use. Make sure that you are using hypoallergenic, non-alcohol, non-scented, and light formulated products. You can also stick to natural treatment like aloe vera.

If you are not inclined to applying anything on your painful patches, cold gels or cold compress through wipes, towels, or bags may also soothe the skin.

- **First timers.** For first timers, the measures above are the same for controlling pain. Additionally, you may want to start waxing in small patches to avoid overwhelming your skin. Make sure you also have enough hair length (not too short, not too long) so that you only have to wax the area once.

Change in skin colour

Generally, waxing is not supposed to cause any skin discoloration. The dark shadowy spots you might observe post wax is probably a consequence of untimely skin exposure. Remember that waxing is capable of also lifting up dead skin cells, which exposes the more sensitive skin layers. This layer can be more sensitive to the sun and might burn after extreme or too much sun exposure.

To avoid any discoloration, make sure to avoid the sun at least 24 hours post- waxing. Also, avoid applying other products that might just irritate and/ or burn the skin eventually causing redness, inflammation, or darkening.

By the time you are ready for the sun, continue the skin care by applying sunblock on the waxed area. It goes without saying that you must also avoid tanning in any way.

If the area has already started darkening and it cannot be helped anymore, you may just consider using skin lighting products instead. These can be in the forms of soap, lotions, and even toners or creams. Again, make sure that the waxed area has first recovered from redness and inflammation (usually at least after 24 hours) before you even put any chemically formulated products on your skin.

TIP: If you need the flawless skin immediately, borrow the power of make-up. You may stick to using a good foundation and/ or use a reliable concealer. We cannot repeat enough that when using any of these products, one must consider the current condition of the skin prior to any application.

Thank you note

It's been a pleasure to write this book for you. I really enjoyed it. Now it's your turn to become an expert at waxing!

Use the troubleshooting tips described in this book to help you along the way. Thanks for reading this book and have a great wax!

Sarah H. Carter